Strain

MW00364965

Grower

Acquired $

| Indica | Hybrid | Sativa |

☐ Flower   ☐ Edible   ☐ Concentrate

Symptoms Relieved

_____

_____

_____

_____

Sweet

Fruity   Floral

Sour   Spicy

Earthy   Herbal

Woodsy

Notes

_____

_____

_____

_____

_____

_____

Effects	Strength				
Peaceful	○	○	○	○	○
Sleepy	○	○	○	○	○
Pain Relief	○	○	○	○	○
Hungry	○	○	○	○	○
Uplifted	○	○	○	○	○
Creative	○	○	○	○	○

Ratings ☆ ☆ ☆ ☆ ☆

Strain

Grower _____   Date _____

Acquired _____ $ _____

| Indica | Hybrid | Sativa |

☐ Flower   ☐ Edible   ☐ Concentrate

Symptoms Relieved

_____

_____

_____

_____

_____

Sweet

Fruity   Floral

Sour   Spicy

Earthy   Herbal

Woodsy

Notes

_____

_____

_____

_____

_____

_____

Effects	**Strength**				
Peaceful	○	○	○	○	○
Sleepy	○	○	○	○	○
Pain Relief	○	○	○	○	○
Hungry	○	○	○	○	○
Uplifted	○	○	○	○	○
Creative	○	○	○	○	○

Ratings ☆ ☆ ☆ ☆ ☆

Strain

Grower _____   Date _____

Acquired _____ $ _____

Indica	Hybrid	Sativa

☐ Flower   ☐ Edible   ☐ Concentrate

Symptoms Relieved

_____

_____

_____

_____

_____

Sweet

Fruity   Floral

Sour   Spicy

Earthy   Herbal

Woodsy

Notes

_____

_____

_____

_____

_____

_____

Effects	Strength				
Peaceful	○	○	○	○	○
Sleepy	○	○	○	○	○
Pain Relief	○	○	○	○	○
Hungry	○	○	○	○	○
Uplifted	○	○	○	○	○
Creative	○	○	○	○	○

Ratings ☆ ☆ ☆ ☆ ☆

Strain

Grower _____ Date _____

Acquired _____ $ _____

| Indica | Hybrid | Sativa |

☐ Flower ☐ Edible ☐ Concentrate

Symptoms Relieved

_____

_____

_____

_____

Sweet

Fruity   Floral

Sour   Spicy

Earthy   Herbal

Woodsy

Notes

_____

_____

_____

_____

_____

_____

Effects	Strength				
Peaceful	○	○	○	○	○
Sleepy	○	○	○	○	○
Pain Relief	○	○	○	○	○
Hungry	○	○	○	○	○
Uplifted	○	○	○	○	○
Creative	○	○	○	○	○

Ratings ☆ ☆ ☆ ☆ ☆

Strain

Grower _____   Date _____

Acquired _____ $ _____

Indica	Hybrid	Sativa

☐ Flower   ☐ Edible   ☐ Concentrate

Symptoms Relieved

_____

_____

_____

_____

_____

Sweet
Fruity   Floral
Sour   Spicy
Earthy   Herbal
Woodsy

Notes

_____

_____

_____

_____

_____

_____

_____

Effects	Strength				
Peaceful	○	○	○	○	○
Sleepy	○	○	○	○	○
Pain Relief	○	○	○	○	○
Hungry	○	○	○	○	○
Uplifted	○	○	○	○	○
Creative	○	○	○	○	○

Ratings ☆ ☆ ☆ ☆ ☆

Strain

Grower _____   Date _____

Acquired _____ $ _____

Indica	Hybrid	Sativa

☐ Flower   ☐ Edible   ☐ Concentrate

Symptoms Relieved

_____

_____

_____

_____

Sweet

Fruity   Floral

Sour   Spicy

Earthy   Herbal

Woodsy

Notes

_____

_____

_____

_____

_____

_____

Effects	Strength				
Peaceful	○	○	○	○	○
Sleepy	○	○	○	○	○
Pain Relief	○	○	○	○	○
Hungry	○	○	○	○	○
Uplifted	○	○	○	○	○
Creative	○	○	○	○	○

Ratings ☆ ☆ ☆ ☆ ☆

Strain

Grower _____ Date _____

Acquired _____ $ _____

| Indica | Hybrid | Sativa |

☐ Flower   ☐ Edible   ☐ Concentrate

Symptoms Relieved

_____

_____

_____

_____

Sweet
Fruity   Floral
Sour   Spicy
Earthy   Herbal
Woodsy

Notes

_____

_____

_____

_____

_____

_____

Effects	Strength				
Peaceful	○	○	○	○	○
Sleepy	○	○	○	○	○
Pain Relief	○	○	○	○	○
Hungry	○	○	○	○	○
Uplifted	○	○	○	○	○
Creative	○	○	○	○	○

Ratings ☆ ☆ ☆ ☆ ☆

Strain

Grower _____   Date _____

Acquired _____ $ _____

Indica	Hybrid	Sativa

☐ Flower   ☐ Edible   ☐ Concentrate

Symptoms Relieved

_____

_____

_____

_____

Sweet
Fruity   Floral
Sour   Spicy
Earthy   Herbal
Woodsy

Notes

_____

_____

_____

_____

_____

_____

Effects	Strength				
Peaceful	○	○	○	○	○
Sleepy	○	○	○	○	○
Pain Relief	○	○	○	○	○
Hungry	○	○	○	○	○
Uplifted	○	○	○	○	○
Creative	○	○	○	○	○

Ratings ☆ ☆ ☆ ☆ ☆

Strain

Grower _____   Date _____

Acquired _____ $ _____

| Indica | Hybrid | Sativa |

☐ Flower   ☐ Edible   ☐ Concentrate

Symptoms Relieved

_____

_____

_____

_____

Sweet

Fruity   Floral

Sour   Spicy

Earthy   Herbal

Woodsy

Notes

_____

_____

_____

_____

_____

_____

Effects	Strength				
Peaceful	○	○	○	○	○
Sleepy	○	○	○	○	○
Pain Relief	○	○	○	○	○
Hungry	○	○	○	○	○
Uplifted	○	○	○	○	○
Creative	○	○	○	○	○

Ratings ☆ ☆ ☆ ☆ ☆

Strain

Grower _____   Date _____

Acquired _____ $ _____

Indica	Hybrid	Sativa

☐ Flower ☐ Edible ☐ Concentrate

Symptoms Relieved

_____

_____

_____

_____

_____

Sweet
Fruity   Floral
Sour   Spicy
Earthy   Herbal
Woodsy

Notes

_____

_____

_____

_____

_____

_____

Effects	Strength				
Peaceful	○	○	○	○	○
Sleepy	○	○	○	○	○
Pain Relief	○	○	○	○	○
Hungry	○	○	○	○	○
Uplifted	○	○	○	○	○
Creative	○	○	○	○	○

Ratings ☆ ☆ ☆ ☆ ☆

Strain

Grower _____   Date _____

Acquired _____ $ _____

| Indica | Hybrid | Sativa |

☐ Flower   ☐ Edible   ☐ Concentrate

Symptoms Relieved

_____

_____

_____

_____

_____

Sweet

Fruity   Floral

Sour   Spicy

Earthy   Herbal

Woodsy

Notes

_____

_____

_____

_____

_____

_____

_____

_____

Effects	Strength				
Peaceful	○	○	○	○	○
Sleepy	○	○	○	○	○
Pain Relief	○	○	○	○	○
Hungry	○	○	○	○	○
Uplifted	○	○	○	○	○
Creative	○	○	○	○	○

Ratings ☆ ☆ ☆ ☆ ☆

Strain

Grower _____ Date _____

Acquired _____ $ _____

Indica	Hybrid	Sativa

☐ Flower ☐ Edible ☐ Concentrate

Symptoms Relieved

_____

_____

_____

_____

Notes

_____

_____

_____

_____

_____

_____

Sweet

Fruity

Floral

Sour

Spicy

Earthy

Herbal

Woodsy

Effects	Strength				
Peaceful	○	○	○	○	○
Sleepy	○	○	○	○	○
Pain Relief	○	○	○	○	○
Hungry	○	○	○	○	○
Uplifted	○	○	○	○	○
Creative	○	○	○	○	○

Ratings ☆ ☆ ☆ ☆ ☆

Strain

Grower _____ Date _____

Acquired _____ $ _____

| Indica | Hybrid | Sativa |

☐ Flower ☐ Edible ☐ Concentrate

Symptoms Relieved

_____
_____
_____
_____

Sweet
Fruity   Floral
Sour   Spicy
Earthy   Herbal
Woodsy

Notes

_____
_____
_____
_____
_____
_____

Effects	Strength				
Peaceful	○	○	○	○	○
Sleepy	○	○	○	○	○
Pain Relief	○	○	○	○	○
Hungry	○	○	○	○	○
Uplifted	○	○	○	○	○
Creative	○	○	○	○	○

Ratings ☆ ☆ ☆ ☆ ☆

Strain

Grower _____   Date _____

Acquired _____ $ _____

Indica	Hybrid	Sativa

☐ Flower   ☐ Edible   ☐ Concentrate

Symptoms Relieved

_____

_____

_____

_____

_____

Sweet

Fruity   Floral

Sour   Spicy

Earthy   Herbal

Woodsy

Notes

_____

_____

_____

_____

_____

_____

_____

Effects	Strength				
Peaceful	○	○	○	○	○
Sleepy	○	○	○	○	○
Pain Relief	○	○	○	○	○
Hungry	○	○	○	○	○
Uplifted	○	○	○	○	○
Creative	○	○	○	○	○

Ratings ☆ ☆ ☆ ☆ ☆

Strain

Grower _____ Date _____

Acquired _____ $ _____

| Indica | Hybrid | Sativa |

☐ Flower ☐ Edible ☐ Concentrate

Symptoms Relieved

_____

_____

_____

_____

_____

Sweet
Fruity   Floral
Sour   Spicy
Earthy   Herbal
Woodsy

Notes

_____

_____

_____

_____

_____

_____

_____

Effects	Strength
Peaceful	○ ○ ○ ○ ○
Sleepy	○ ○ ○ ○ ○
Pain Relief	○ ○ ○ ○ ○
Hungry	○ ○ ○ ○ ○
Uplifted	○ ○ ○ ○ ○
Creative	○ ○ ○ ○ ○

Ratings ☆ ☆ ☆ ☆ ☆

Strain

Grower _____   Date _____

Acquired _____ $ _____

| Indica | Hybrid | Sativa |

☐ Flower   ☐ Edible   ☐ Concentrate

Symptoms Relieved

_____

_____

_____

_____

_____

Sweet

Fruity   Floral

Sour   Spicy

Earthy   Herbal

Woodsy

Notes

_____

_____

_____

_____

_____

_____

Effects	Strength				
Peaceful	○	○	○	○	○
Sleepy	○	○	○	○	○
Pain Relief	○	○	○	○	○
Hungry	○	○	○	○	○
Uplifted	○	○	○	○	○
Creative	○	○	○	○	○

Ratings ☆ ☆ ☆ ☆ ☆

Strain

Grower _____ Date _____

Acquired _____ $ _____

Indica	Hybrid	Sativa

☐ Flower ☐ Edible ☐ Concentrate

Symptoms Relieved

_____
_____
_____
_____

Sweet
Fruity
Floral
Sour
Spicy
Earthy
Herbal
Woodsy

Notes

_____
_____
_____
_____
_____
_____

Effects	Strength				
Peaceful	○	○	○	○	○
Sleepy	○	○	○	○	○
Pain Relief	○	○	○	○	○
Hungry	○	○	○	○	○
Uplifted	○	○	○	○	○
Creative	○	○	○	○	○

Ratings ☆ ☆ ☆ ☆ ☆

Strain

Grower _____   Date _____

Acquired _____ $ _____

Indica	Hybrid	Sativa

☐ Flower   ☐ Edible   ☐ Concentrate

Symptoms Relieved

_____

_____

_____

_____

Sweet

Fruity

Floral

Sour

Spicy

Earthy

Herbal

Woodsy

Notes

_____

_____

_____

_____

_____

_____

Effects	Strength				
Peaceful	○	○	○	○	○
Sleepy	○	○	○	○	○
Pain Relief	○	○	○	○	○
Hungry	○	○	○	○	○
Uplifted	○	○	○	○	○
Creative	○	○	○	○	○

Ratings ☆ ☆ ☆ ☆ ☆

Strain

Grower _____ Date _____

Acquired _____ $ _____

| Indica | Hybrid | Sativa |

☐ Flower ☐ Edible ☐ Concentrate

Symptoms Relieved

_____

_____

_____

_____

Sweet

Fruity   Floral

Sour   Spicy

Earthy   Herbal

Woodsy

Notes

_____

_____

_____

_____

_____

_____

Effects	Strength				
Peaceful	○	○	○	○	○
Sleepy	○	○	○	○	○
Pain Relief	○	○	○	○	○
Hungry	○	○	○	○	○
Uplifted	○	○	○	○	○
Creative	○	○	○	○	○

Ratings ☆ ☆ ☆ ☆ ☆

Strain

Grower _____ Date _____

Acquired _____ $ _____

| Indica | Hybrid | Sativa |

☐ Flower   ☐ Edible   ☐ Concentrate

Symptoms Relieved

_____
_____
_____
_____
_____

Sweet
Fruity   Floral
Sour   Spicy
Earthy   Herbal
Woodsy

Notes

_____
_____
_____
_____
_____
_____

Effects	Strength
Peaceful	○ ○ ○ ○ ○
Sleepy	○ ○ ○ ○ ○
Pain Relief	○ ○ ○ ○ ○
Hungry	○ ○ ○ ○ ○
Uplifted	○ ○ ○ ○ ○
Creative	○ ○ ○ ○ ○

Ratings ☆ ☆ ☆ ☆ ☆

Strain

Grower _____   Date _____

Acquired _____ $ _____

Indica	Hybrid	Sativa

☐ Flower   ☐ Edible   ☐ Concentrate

Symptoms Relieved

_____
_____
_____
_____
_____

Sweet
Fruity   Floral
Sour   Spicy
Earthy   Herbal
Woodsy

Notes

_____
_____
_____
_____
_____
_____

Effects	Strength				
Peaceful	○	○	○	○	○
Sleepy	○	○	○	○	○
Pain Relief	○	○	○	○	○
Hungry	○	○	○	○	○
Uplifted	○	○	○	○	○
Creative	○	○	○	○	○

Ratings ☆ ☆ ☆ ☆ ☆

Strain

Grower _____ Date _____

Acquired _____ $ _____

| Indica | Hybrid | Sativa |

☐ Flower   ☐ Edible   ☐ Concentrate

Symptoms Relieved

_____

_____

_____

_____

Sweet
Fruity   Floral
Sour   Spicy
Earthy   Herbal
Woodsy

Notes

_____

_____

_____

_____

_____

_____

Effects	Strength				
Peaceful	○	○	○	○	○
Sleepy	○	○	○	○	○
Pain Relief	○	○	○	○	○
Hungry	○	○	○	○	○
Uplifted	○	○	○	○	○
Creative	○	○	○	○	○

Ratings ☆ ☆ ☆ ☆ ☆

Strain

Grower _____ Date _____

Acquired _____ $ _____

Indica	Hybrid	Sativa

☐ Flower ☐ Edible ☐ Concentrate

Symptoms Relieved

_____

_____

_____

_____

Sweet

Fruity   Floral

Sour   Spicy

Earthy   Herbal

Woodsy

Notes

_____

_____

_____

_____

_____

_____

Effects	Strength				
Peaceful	○	○	○	○	○
Sleepy	○	○	○	○	○
Pain Relief	○	○	○	○	○
Hungry	○	○	○	○	○
Uplifted	○	○	○	○	○
Creative	○	○	○	○	○

Ratings ☆ ☆ ☆ ☆ ☆

Strain

Grower _____   Date _____

Acquired _____ $ _____

| Indica | Hybrid | Sativa |

☐ Flower ☐ Edible ☐ Concentrate

Symptoms Relieved

_____

_____

_____

_____

_____

Sweet

Fruity   Floral

Sour   Spicy

Earthy   Herbal

Woodsy

Notes

_____

_____

_____

_____

_____

_____

Effects	**Strength**				
Peaceful	○	○	○	○	○
Sleepy	○	○	○	○	○
Pain Relief	○	○	○	○	○
Hungry	○	○	○	○	○
Uplifted	○	○	○	○	○
Creative	○	○	○	○	○

Ratings ☆ ☆ ☆ ☆ ☆

Strain

Grower _____ Date _____

Acquired _____ $ _____

| Indica | Hybrid | Sativa |

☐ Flower ☐ Edible ☐ Concentrate

Symptoms Relieved

_____

_____

_____

_____

Sweet

Fruity   Floral

Sour   Spicy

Earthy   Herbal

Woodsy

Notes

_____

_____

_____

_____

_____

_____

Effects	Strength				
Peaceful	○	○	○	○	○
Sleepy	○	○	○	○	○
Pain Relief	○	○	○	○	○
Hungry	○	○	○	○	○
Uplifted	○	○	○	○	○
Creative	○	○	○	○	○

Ratings ☆ ☆ ☆ ☆ ☆

Strain

Grower _____   Date _____

Acquired _____ $ _____

Indica	Hybrid	Sativa

☐ Flower   ☐ Edible   ☐ Concentrate

Symptoms Relieved

_____

_____

_____

_____

_____

Sweet
Fruity   Floral
Sour   Spicy
Earthy   Herbal
Woodsy

Notes

_____

_____

_____

_____

_____

_____

Effects	Strength				
Peaceful	○	○	○	○	○
Sleepy	○	○	○	○	○
Pain Relief	○	○	○	○	○
Hungry	○	○	○	○	○
Uplifted	○	○	○	○	○
Creative	○	○	○	○	○

Ratings ☆ ☆ ☆ ☆ ☆

Strain

Grower _____ Date _____

Acquired _____ $ _____

| Indica | Hybrid | Sativa |

☐ Flower ☐ Edible ☐ Concentrate

Symptoms Relieved

_____

_____

_____

_____

_____

Sweet

Fruity / Floral

Sour / Spicy

Earthy / Herbal

Woodsy

Notes

_____

_____

_____

_____

_____

_____

Effects	Strength				
Peaceful	○	○	○	○	○
Sleepy	○	○	○	○	○
Pain Relief	○	○	○	○	○
Hungry	○	○	○	○	○
Uplifted	○	○	○	○	○
Creative	○	○	○	○	○

Ratings ☆ ☆ ☆ ☆ ☆

Strain

Grower _____ Date _____

Acquired _____ $ _____

Indica	Hybrid	Sativa

☐ Flower　☐ Edible　☐ Concentrate

Symptoms Relieved

_____

_____

_____

_____

Sweet

Fruity ・ Floral

Sour ・ Spicy

Earthy ・ Herbal

Woodsy

Notes

_____

_____

_____

_____

_____

_____

Effects	Strength				
Peaceful	○	○	○	○	○
Sleepy	○	○	○	○	○
Pain Relief	○	○	○	○	○
Hungry	○	○	○	○	○
Uplifted	○	○	○	○	○
Creative	○	○	○	○	○

Ratings ☆ ☆ ☆ ☆ ☆

Strain

Grower _____   Date _____

Acquired _____ $ _____

Indica	Hybrid	Sativa

☐ Flower   ☐ Edible   ☐ Concentrate

Symptoms Relieved

_____

_____

_____

_____

_____

Sweet

Fruity   Floral

Sour   Spicy

Earthy   Herbal

Woodsy

Notes

_____

_____

_____

_____

_____

_____

_____

Effects	Strength				
Peaceful	○	○	○	○	○
Sleepy	○	○	○	○	○
Pain Relief	○	○	○	○	○
Hungry	○	○	○	○	○
Uplifted	○	○	○	○	○
Creative	○	○	○	○	○

Ratings ☆ ☆ ☆ ☆ ☆

Strain

Grower _____   Date _____

Acquired _____ $ _____

| Indica | Hybrid | Sativa |

☐ Flower   ☐ Edible   ☐ Concentrate

Symptoms Relieved

_____

_____

_____

_____

_____

Sweet

Fruity   Floral

Sour   Spicy

Earthy   Herbal

Woodsy

Notes

_____

_____

_____

_____

_____

Effects	Strength				
Peaceful	○	○	○	○	○
Sleepy	○	○	○	○	○
Pain Relief	○	○	○	○	○
Hungry	○	○	○	○	○
Uplifted	○	○	○	○	○
Creative	○	○	○	○	○

Ratings ☆ ☆ ☆ ☆ ☆

Strain

Grower _____ Date _____

Acquired _____ $ _____

| Indica | Hybrid | Sativa |

☐ Flower   ☐ Edible   ☐ Concentrate

Symptoms Relieved

_____

_____

_____

_____

Sweet

Fruity   Floral

Sour   Spicy

Earthy   Herbal

Woodsy

Notes

_____

_____

_____

_____

_____

_____

Effects	Strength				
Peaceful	○	○	○	○	○
Sleepy	○	○	○	○	○
Pain Relief	○	○	○	○	○
Hungry	○	○	○	○	○
Uplifted	○	○	○	○	○
Creative	○	○	○	○	○

Ratings ☆ ☆ ☆ ☆ ☆

Strain

Grower _____ Date _____

Acquired _____ $ _____

| Indica | Hybrid | Sativa |

☐ Flower ☐ Edible ☐ Concentrate

Symptoms Relieved

_____

_____

_____

_____

_____

Sweet
Fruity   Floral
Sour   Spicy
Earthy   Herbal
Woodsy

Notes

_____

_____

_____

_____

_____

Effects	Strength				
Peaceful	○	○	○	○	○
Sleepy	○	○	○	○	○
Pain Relief	○	○	○	○	○
Hungry	○	○	○	○	○
Uplifted	○	○	○	○	○
Creative	○	○	○	○	○

Ratings ☆ ☆ ☆ ☆ ☆

Strain

Grower _____ Date _____

Acquired _____ $ _____

Indica	Hybrid	Sativa

☐ Flower ☐ Edible ☐ Concentrate

Symptoms Relieved

_____

_____

_____

_____

Sweet
Fruity   Floral
Sour   Spicy
Earthy   Herbal
Woodsy

Notes

_____

_____

_____

_____

_____

Effects	Strength				
Peaceful	○	○	○	○	○
Sleepy	○	○	○	○	○
Pain Relief	○	○	○	○	○
Hungry	○	○	○	○	○
Uplifted	○	○	○	○	○
Creative	○	○	○	○	○

Ratings ☆ ☆ ☆ ☆ ☆

Strain

Grower _____ Date _____

Acquired _____ $ _____

Indica	Hybrid	Sativa

☐ Flower   ☐ Edible   ☐ Concentrate

Symptoms Relieved

_____

_____

_____

_____

Sweet / Fruity / Floral / Sour / Spicy / Earthy / Herbal / Woodsy

Notes

_____

_____

_____

_____

_____

_____

Effects	Strength				
Peaceful	○	○	○	○	○
Sleepy	○	○	○	○	○
Pain Relief	○	○	○	○	○
Hungry	○	○	○	○	○
Uplifted	○	○	○	○	○
Creative	○	○	○	○	○

Ratings ☆ ☆ ☆ ☆ ☆

Strain

Grower _____ Date _____

Acquired _____ $ _____

Indica	Hybrid	Sativa

☐ Flower ☐ Edible ☐ Concentrate

Symptoms Relieved

_____

_____

_____

_____

Sweet
Fruity   Floral
Sour   Spicy
Earthy   Herbal
Woodsy

Notes

_____

_____

_____

_____

_____

_____

Effects	Strength				
Peaceful	○	○	○	○	○
Sleepy	○	○	○	○	○
Pain Relief	○	○	○	○	○
Hungry	○	○	○	○	○
Uplifted	○	○	○	○	○
Creative	○	○	○	○	○

Ratings ☆ ☆ ☆ ☆ ☆

Strain

Grower _____   Date _____

Acquired _____ $ _____

Indica	Hybrid	Sativa

☐ Flower ☐ Edible ☐ Concentrate

Symptoms Relieved

_____

_____

_____

_____

_____

Sweet

Fruity

Floral

Sour

Spicy

Earthy

Herbal

Woodsy

Notes

_____

_____

_____

_____

_____

_____

_____

Effects	Strength				
Peaceful	○	○	○	○	○
Sleepy	○	○	○	○	○
Pain Relief	○	○	○	○	○
Hungry	○	○	○	○	○
Uplifted	○	○	○	○	○
Creative	○	○	○	○	○

Ratings ☆ ☆ ☆ ☆ ☆

Strain

Grower _____   Date _____

Acquired _____ $ _____

Indica	Hybrid	Sativa

☐ Flower   ☐ Edible   ☐ Concentrate

Symptoms Relieved

_____

_____

_____

_____

_____

Sweet

Fruity   Floral

Sour   Spicy

Earthy   Herbal

Woodsy

Notes

_____

_____

_____

_____

_____

_____

Effects	Strength				
Peaceful	○	○	○	○	○
Sleepy	○	○	○	○	○
Pain Relief	○	○	○	○	○
Hungry	○	○	○	○	○
Uplifted	○	○	○	○	○
Creative	○	○	○	○	○

Ratings ☆ ☆ ☆ ☆ ☆

Strain

Grower _____   Date _____

Acquired _____ $ _____

Indica	Hybrid	Sativa

☐ Flower   ☐ Edible   ☐ Concentrate

Symptoms Relieved

_____

_____

_____

_____

Sweet

Fruity   Floral

Sour   Spicy

Earthy   Herbal

Woodsy

Notes

_____

_____

_____

_____

_____

_____

Effects	Strength				
Peaceful	○	○	○	○	○
Sleepy	○	○	○	○	○
Pain Relief	○	○	○	○	○
Hungry	○	○	○	○	○
Uplifted	○	○	○	○	○
Creative	○	○	○	○	○

Ratings ☆ ☆ ☆ ☆ ☆

Strain

Grower _____ Date _____

Acquired _____ $ _____

Indica	Hybrid	Sativa

☐ Flower ☐ Edible ☐ Concentrate

Symptoms Relieved

_____

_____

_____

_____

_____

Sweet
Fruity   Floral
Sour   Spicy
Earthy   Herbal
Woodsy

Notes

_____

_____

_____

_____

_____

_____

_____

Effects	Strength				
Peaceful	○	○	○	○	○
Sleepy	○	○	○	○	○
Pain Relief	○	○	○	○	○
Hungry	○	○	○	○	○
Uplifted	○	○	○	○	○
Creative	○	○	○	○	○

Ratings ☆ ☆ ☆ ☆ ☆

Strain

Grower _____   Date _____

Acquired _____ $ _____

| Indica | Hybrid | Sativa |

☐ Flower ☐ Edible ☐ Concentrate

Symptoms Relieved

_____

_____

_____

_____

_____

Sweet

Fruity   Floral

Sour   Spicy

Earthy   Herbal

Woodsy

Notes

_____

_____

_____

_____

_____

_____

Effects	Strength				
Peaceful	○	○	○	○	○
Sleepy	○	○	○	○	○
Pain Relief	○	○	○	○	○
Hungry	○	○	○	○	○
Uplifted	○	○	○	○	○
Creative	○	○	○	○	○

Ratings ☆ ☆ ☆ ☆ ☆

Strain

Grower _____   Date _____

Acquired _____ $ _____

| Indica | Hybrid | Sativa |

☐ Flower   ☐ Edible   ☐ Concentrate

Symptoms Relieved

_____

_____

_____

_____

Sweet
Fruity   Floral
Sour   Spicy
Earthy   Herbal
Woodsy

Notes

_____

_____

_____

_____

_____

_____

Effects	Strength
Peaceful	○ ○ ○ ○ ○
Sleepy	○ ○ ○ ○ ○
Pain Relief	○ ○ ○ ○ ○
Hungry	○ ○ ○ ○ ○
Uplifted	○ ○ ○ ○ ○
Creative	○ ○ ○ ○ ○

Ratings ☆ ☆ ☆ ☆ ☆

Strain

Grower _____   Date _____

Acquired _____ $ _____

| Indica | Hybrid | Sativa |

☐ Flower   ☐ Edible   ☐ Concentrate

Symptoms Relieved

_____

_____

_____

_____

Sweet
Fruity   Floral
Sour   Spicy
Earthy   Herbal
Woodsy

Notes

_____

_____

_____

_____

_____

Effects	Strength				
Peaceful	○	○	○	○	○
Sleepy	○	○	○	○	○
Pain Relief	○	○	○	○	○
Hungry	○	○	○	○	○
Uplifted	○	○	○	○	○
Creative	○	○	○	○	○

Ratings ☆ ☆ ☆ ☆ ☆

Strain

Grower _____ Date _____

Acquired _____ $ _____

| Indica | Hybrid | Sativa |

☐ Flower   ☐ Edible   ☐ Concentrate

Symptoms Relieved

_____

_____

_____

_____

_____

Sweet

Fruity   Floral

Sour   Spicy

Earthy   Herbal

Woodsy

Notes

_____

_____

_____

_____

_____

_____

Effects	Strength
Peaceful	○ ○ ○ ○ ○
Sleepy	○ ○ ○ ○ ○
Pain Relief	○ ○ ○ ○ ○
Hungry	○ ○ ○ ○ ○
Uplifted	○ ○ ○ ○ ○
Creative	○ ○ ○ ○ ○

Ratings ☆ ☆ ☆ ☆ ☆

Strain

Grower _____   Date _____

Acquired _____ $ _____

| Indica | Hybrid | Sativa |

☐ Flower   ☐ Edible   ☐ Concentrate

Symptoms Relieved

_____

_____

_____

_____

_____

Sweet

Fruity   Floral

Sour   Spicy

Earthy   Herbal

Woodsy

Notes

_____

_____

_____

_____

_____

_____

Effects	**Strength**				
Peaceful	○	○	○	○	○
Sleepy	○	○	○	○	○
Pain Relief	○	○	○	○	○
Hungry	○	○	○	○	○
Uplifted	○	○	○	○	○
Creative	○	○	○	○	○

Ratings ☆ ☆ ☆ ☆ ☆

Strain

Grower _____   Date _____

Acquired _____ $ _____

| Indica | Hybrid | Sativa |

☐ Flower   ☐ Edible   ☐ Concentrate

Symptoms Relieved

_____
_____
_____
_____

Sweet

Fruity   Floral

Sour   Spicy

Earthy   Herbal

Woodsy

Notes

_____
_____
_____
_____
_____
_____

Effects	Strength				
Peaceful	○	○	○	○	○
Sleepy	○	○	○	○	○
Pain Relief	○	○	○	○	○
Hungry	○	○	○	○	○
Uplifted	○	○	○	○	○
Creative	○	○	○	○	○

Ratings ☆ ☆ ☆ ☆ ☆

Strain

Grower _____   Date _____

Acquired _____ $ _____

Indica	Hybrid	Sativa

☐ Flower   ☐ Edible   ☐ Concentrate

Symptoms Relieved

_____

_____

_____

_____

_____

Sweet
Fruity   Floral
Sour   Spicy
Earthy   Herbal
Woodsy

Notes

_____

_____

_____

_____

_____

_____

Effects	Strength				
Peaceful	○	○	○	○	○
Sleepy	○	○	○	○	○
Pain Relief	○	○	○	○	○
Hungry	○	○	○	○	○
Uplifted	○	○	○	○	○
Creative	○	○	○	○	○

Ratings ☆ ☆ ☆ ☆ ☆

Strain

Grower _____   Date _____

Acquired _____ $ _____

| Indica | Hybrid | Sativa |

☐ Flower ☐ Edible ☐ Concentrate

Symptoms Relieved

_____

_____

_____

_____

Sweet · Floral · Spicy · Herbal · Woodsy · Earthy · Sour · Fruity

Notes

_____

_____

_____

_____

_____

_____

Effects	Strength				
Peaceful	○	○	○	○	○
Sleepy	○	○	○	○	○
Pain Relief	○	○	○	○	○
Hungry	○	○	○	○	○
Uplifted	○	○	○	○	○
Creative	○	○	○	○	○

Ratings ☆ ☆ ☆ ☆ ☆

Strain

Grower _____   Date _____

Acquired _____ $ _____

| Indica | Hybrid | Sativa |

☐ Flower   ☐ Edible   ☐ Concentrate

Symptoms Relieved

_____
_____
_____
_____
_____

Sweet

Fruity   Floral

Sour   Spicy

Earthy   Herbal

Woodsy

Notes

_____
_____
_____
_____
_____
_____
_____

Effects	Strength
Peaceful	○ ○ ○ ○ ○
Sleepy	○ ○ ○ ○ ○
Pain Relief	○ ○ ○ ○ ○
Hungry	○ ○ ○ ○ ○
Uplifted	○ ○ ○ ○ ○
Creative	○ ○ ○ ○ ○

Ratings ☆ ☆ ☆ ☆ ☆

Strain

Grower _____ Date _____

Acquired _____ $ _____

Indica	Hybrid	Sativa

☐ Flower ☐ Edible ☐ Concentrate

Symptoms Relieved

_____

_____

_____

_____

Sweet
Fruity   Floral
Sour   Spicy
Earthy   Herbal
Woodsy

Notes

_____

_____

_____

_____

_____

Effects	Strength				
Peaceful	○	○	○	○	○
Sleepy	○	○	○	○	○
Pain Relief	○	○	○	○	○
Hungry	○	○	○	○	○
Uplifted	○	○	○	○	○
Creative	○	○	○	○	○

Ratings ☆ ☆ ☆ ☆ ☆

Strain

Grower _____ Date _____

Acquired _____ $ _____

| Indica | Hybrid | Sativa |

☐ Flower ☐ Edible ☐ Concentrate

Symptoms Relieved

_____

_____

_____

_____

_____

Sweet
Fruity   Floral
Sour   Spicy
Earthy   Herbal
Woodsy

Notes

_____

_____

_____

_____

_____

_____

Effects	Strength				
Peaceful	○	○	○	○	○
Sleepy	○	○	○	○	○
Pain Relief	○	○	○	○	○
Hungry	○	○	○	○	○
Uplifted	○	○	○	○	○
Creative	○	○	○	○	○

Ratings ☆ ☆ ☆ ☆ ☆

Strain

Grower _____ Date _____

Acquired _____ $ _____

Indica	Hybrid	Sativa

☐ Flower ☐ Edible ☐ Concentrate

Symptoms Relieved

_____

_____

_____

_____

Sweet

Fruity   Floral

Sour   Spicy

Earthy   Herbal

Woodsy

Notes

_____

_____

_____

_____

_____

_____

Effects	Strength				
Peaceful	○	○	○	○	○
Sleepy	○	○	○	○	○
Pain Relief	○	○	○	○	○
Hungry	○	○	○	○	○
Uplifted	○	○	○	○	○
Creative	○	○	○	○	○

Ratings ☆ ☆ ☆ ☆ ☆

Strain

Grower _____ Date _____

Acquired _____ $ _____

Indica	Hybrid	Sativa

☐ Flower ☐ Edible ☐ Concentrate

Symptoms Relieved

_____

_____

_____

_____

_____

Sweet
Fruity   Floral
Sour   Spicy
Earthy   Herbal
Woodsy

Notes

_____

_____

_____

_____

_____

_____

Effects	Strength				
Peaceful	○	○	○	○	○
Sleepy	○	○	○	○	○
Pain Relief	○	○	○	○	○
Hungry	○	○	○	○	○
Uplifted	○	○	○	○	○
Creative	○	○	○	○	○

Ratings ☆ ☆ ☆ ☆ ☆

Strain

Grower _____   Date _____

Acquired _____ $ _____

| Indica | Hybrid | Sativa |

☐ Flower   ☐ Edible   ☐ Concentrate

Symptoms Relieved

_____

_____

_____

_____

_____

Sweet
Fruity   Floral

Sour   Spicy

Earthy   Herbal

Woodsy

Notes

_____

_____

_____

_____

_____

_____

_____

Effects	Strength				
Peaceful	○	○	○	○	○
Sleepy	○	○	○	○	○
Pain Relief	○	○	○	○	○
Hungry	○	○	○	○	○
Uplifted	○	○	○	○	○
Creative	○	○	○	○	○

Ratings ☆ ☆ ☆ ☆ ☆

Strain

Grower _____   Date _____

Acquired _____ $ _____

| Indica | Hybrid | Sativa |

☐ Flower   ☐ Edible   ☐ Concentrate

Symptoms Relieved

_____
_____
_____
_____
_____

Sweet
Fruity   Floral
Sour   Spicy
Earthy   Herbal
Woodsy

Notes

_____
_____
_____
_____
_____
_____

Effects	Strength
Peaceful	○ ○ ○ ○ ○
Sleepy	○ ○ ○ ○ ○
Pain Relief	○ ○ ○ ○ ○
Hungry	○ ○ ○ ○ ○
Uplifted	○ ○ ○ ○ ○
Creative	○ ○ ○ ○ ○

Ratings ☆ ☆ ☆ ☆ ☆

Strain

Grower _____   Date _____

Acquired _____ $ _____

| Indica | Hybrid | Sativa |

☐ Flower   ☐ Edible   ☐ Concentrate

Symptoms Relieved

_____
_____
_____
_____
_____

Sweet

Fruity   Floral

Sour   Spicy

Earthy   Herbal

Woodsy

Notes

_____
_____
_____
_____
_____
_____

Effects	Strength
Peaceful	○ ○ ○ ○ ○
Sleepy	○ ○ ○ ○ ○
Pain Relief	○ ○ ○ ○ ○
Hungry	○ ○ ○ ○ ○
Uplifted	○ ○ ○ ○ ○
Creative	○ ○ ○ ○ ○

Ratings ☆ ☆ ☆ ☆ ☆

Strain

Grower _____   Date _____

Acquired _____ $ _____

Indica	Hybrid	Sativa

☐ Flower   ☐ Edible   ☐ Concentrate

Symptoms Relieved

_____

_____

_____

_____

_____

Sweet
Fruity   Floral
Sour   Spicy
Earthy   Herbal
Woodsy

Notes

_____

_____

_____

_____

_____

_____

Effects	Strength				
Peaceful	○	○	○	○	○
Sleepy	○	○	○	○	○
Pain Relief	○	○	○	○	○
Hungry	○	○	○	○	○
Uplifted	○	○	○	○	○
Creative	○	○	○	○	○

Ratings ☆ ☆ ☆ ☆ ☆

Strain

Grower _____   Date _____

Acquired _____ $ _____

| Indica | Hybrid | Sativa |

☐ Flower   ☐ Edible   ☐ Concentrate

Symptoms Relieved

_____

_____

_____

_____

Sweet
Fruity   Floral
Sour   Spicy
Earthy   Herbal
Woodsy

Notes

_____

_____

_____

_____

_____

_____

Effects	Strength				
Peaceful	○	○	○	○	○
Sleepy	○	○	○	○	○
Pain Relief	○	○	○	○	○
Hungry	○	○	○	○	○
Uplifted	○	○	○	○	○
Creative	○	○	○	○	○

Ratings ☆ ☆ ☆ ☆ ☆

Strain

Grower _____ Date _____

Acquired _____ $ _____

| Indica | Hybrid | Sativa |

☐ Flower ☐ Edible ☐ Concentrate

Symptoms Relieved

_____
_____
_____
_____

Sweet
Fruity   Floral
Sour   Spicy
Earthy   Herbal
Woodsy

Notes

_____
_____
_____
_____
_____
_____

Effects	Strength				
Peaceful	○	○	○	○	○
Sleepy	○	○	○	○	○
Pain Relief	○	○	○	○	○
Hungry	○	○	○	○	○
Uplifted	○	○	○	○	○
Creative	○	○	○	○	○

Ratings ☆ ☆ ☆ ☆ ☆

Strain

Grower _____   Date _____

Acquired _____ $ _____

| Indica | Hybrid | Sativa |

☐ Flower   ☐ Edible   ☐ Concentrate

Symptoms Relieved

_____

_____

_____

_____

Sweet

Fruity   Floral

Sour   Spicy

Earthy   Herbal

Woodsy

Notes

_____

_____

_____

_____

_____

Effects	Strength				
Peaceful	○	○	○	○	○
Sleepy	○	○	○	○	○
Pain Relief	○	○	○	○	○
Hungry	○	○	○	○	○
Uplifted	○	○	○	○	○
Creative	○	○	○	○	○

Ratings ☆ ☆ ☆ ☆ ☆

Strain

Grower _____ Date _____

Acquired _____ $ _____

Indica	Hybrid	Sativa

☐ Flower ☐ Edible ☐ Concentrate

Symptoms Relieved

_____
_____
_____
_____
_____

Sweet

Fruity Floral

Sour Spicy

Earthy Herbal

Woodsy

Notes

_____
_____
_____
_____
_____
_____

Effects	Strength				
Peaceful	○	○	○	○	○
Sleepy	○	○	○	○	○
Pain Relief	○	○	○	○	○
Hungry	○	○	○	○	○
Uplifted	○	○	○	○	○
Creative	○	○	○	○	○

Ratings ☆ ☆ ☆ ☆ ☆

Strain

Grower _____   Date _____

Acquired _____ $ _____

Indica	Hybrid	Sativa

☐ Flower   ☐ Edible   ☐ Concentrate

Symptoms Relieved

_____

_____

_____

_____

Sweet

Fruity   Floral

Sour   Spicy

Earthy   Herbal

Woodsy

Notes

_____

_____

_____

_____

_____

_____

Effects	Strength				
Peaceful	○	○	○	○	○
Sleepy	○	○	○	○	○
Pain Relief	○	○	○	○	○
Hungry	○	○	○	○	○
Uplifted	○	○	○	○	○
Creative	○	○	○	○	○

Ratings ☆ ☆ ☆ ☆ ☆

Strain

Grower _____ Date _____

Acquired _____ $ _____

| Indica | Hybrid | Sativa |

☐ Flower ☐ Edible ☐ Concentrate

Symptoms Relieved

_____

_____

_____

_____

Sweet
Fruity
Floral
Sour
Spicy
Earthy
Herbal
Woodsy

Notes

_____

_____

_____

_____

_____

_____

Effects	**Strength**				
Peaceful	○	○	○	○	○
Sleepy	○	○	○	○	○
Pain Relief	○	○	○	○	○
Hungry	○	○	○	○	○
Uplifted	○	○	○	○	○
Creative	○	○	○	○	○

Ratings ☆ ☆ ☆ ☆ ☆

Strain

Grower _____ Date _____

Acquired _____ $ _____

| Indica | Hybrid | Sativa |

☐ Flower   ☐ Edible   ☐ Concentrate

Symptoms Relieved

_____

_____

_____

_____

                    Sweet
        Fruity   Floral

    Sour   Spicy

        Earthy   Herbal
                    Woodsy

Notes

_____

_____

_____

_____

_____

_____

Effects	Strength				
Peaceful	○	○	○	○	○
Sleepy	○	○	○	○	○
Pain Relief	○	○	○	○	○
Hungry	○	○	○	○	○
Uplifted	○	○	○	○	○
Creative	○	○	○	○	○

Ratings ☆ ☆ ☆ ☆ ☆

Strain

Grower _____   Date _____

Acquired _____ $ _____

Indica	Hybrid	Sativa

☐ Flower   ☐ Edible   ☐ Concentrate

Symptoms Relieved

_____
_____
_____
_____

Sweet
Fruity   Floral
Sour   Spicy
Earthy   Herbal
Woodsy

Notes

_____
_____
_____
_____
_____
_____

Effects	Strength
Peaceful	○ ○ ○ ○ ○
Sleepy	○ ○ ○ ○ ○
Pain Relief	○ ○ ○ ○ ○
Hungry	○ ○ ○ ○ ○
Uplifted	○ ○ ○ ○ ○
Creative	○ ○ ○ ○ ○

Ratings ☆ ☆ ☆ ☆ ☆

Strain

Grower _____ Date _____

Acquired _____ $ _____

| Indica | Hybrid | Sativa |

☐ Flower ☐ Edible ☐ Concentrate

Symptoms Relieved

_____

_____

_____

_____

_____

Sweet
Fruity   Floral
Sour   Spicy
Earthy   Herbal
Woodsy

Notes

_____

_____

_____

_____

_____

_____

Effects	Strength				
Peaceful	○	○	○	○	○
Sleepy	○	○	○	○	○
Pain Relief	○	○	○	○	○
Hungry	○	○	○	○	○
Uplifted	○	○	○	○	○
Creative	○	○	○	○	○

Ratings ☆ ☆ ☆ ☆ ☆

Strain

Grower _____ Date _____

Acquired _____ $ _____

| Indica | Hybrid | Sativa |

☐ Flower ☐ Edible ☐ Concentrate

Symptoms Relieved

_____
_____
_____
_____

Flavor wheel labels: Sweet, Floral, Spicy, Herbal, Woodsy, Earthy, Sour, Fruity

Notes

_____
_____
_____
_____
_____
_____

Effects	Strength				
Peaceful	○	○	○	○	○
Sleepy	○	○	○	○	○
Pain Relief	○	○	○	○	○
Hungry	○	○	○	○	○
Uplifted	○	○	○	○	○
Creative	○	○	○	○	○

Ratings ☆ ☆ ☆ ☆ ☆

Strain

Grower _____ Date _____

Acquired _____ $ _____

| Indica | Hybrid | Sativa |

☐ Flower   ☐ Edible   ☐ Concentrate

Symptoms Relieved

_____

_____

_____

_____

Sweet

Fruity   Floral

Sour   Spicy

Earthy   Herbal

Woodsy

Notes

_____

_____

_____

_____

_____

Effects	Strength				
Peaceful	○	○	○	○	○
Sleepy	○	○	○	○	○
Pain Relief	○	○	○	○	○
Hungry	○	○	○	○	○
Uplifted	○	○	○	○	○
Creative	○	○	○	○	○

Ratings ☆ ☆ ☆ ☆ ☆

Strain

Grower _____   Date _____

Acquired _____ $ _____

Indica	Hybrid	Sativa

☐ Flower   ☐ Edible   ☐ Concentrate

Symptoms Relieved

_____

_____

_____

_____

Sweet
Fruity   Floral
Sour   Spicy
Earthy   Herbal
Woodsy

Effects	Strength				
Peaceful	○	○	○	○	○
Sleepy	○	○	○	○	○
Pain Relief	○	○	○	○	○
Hungry	○	○	○	○	○
Uplifted	○	○	○	○	○
Creative	○	○	○	○	○

Notes

_____

_____

_____

_____

_____

_____

Ratings ☆ ☆ ☆ ☆ ☆

Strain

Grower _____ Date _____

Acquired _____ $ _____

Indica	Hybrid	Sativa

☐ Flower ☐ Edible ☐ Concentrate

Symptoms Relieved

_____

_____

_____

_____

_____

Sweet

Fruity　　　　　　Floral

Sour　　　　　　　Spicy

Earthy　　　　　　Herbal

Woodsy

Notes

_____

_____

_____

_____

_____

_____

Effects	Strength				
Peaceful	○	○	○	○	○
Sleepy	○	○	○	○	○
Pain Relief	○	○	○	○	○
Hungry	○	○	○	○	○
Uplifted	○	○	○	○	○
Creative	○	○	○	○	○

Ratings ☆ ☆ ☆ ☆ ☆

Strain

Grower _____   Date _____

Acquired _____ $ _____

Indica	Hybrid	Sativa

☐ Flower   ☐ Edible   ☐ Concentrate

Symptoms Relieved

_____

_____

_____

_____

_____

Sweet
Fruity   Floral
Sour   Spicy
Earthy   Herbal
Woodsy

Notes

_____

_____

_____

_____

_____

_____

_____

Effects	Strength				
Peaceful	○	○	○	○	○
Sleepy	○	○	○	○	○
Pain Relief	○	○	○	○	○
Hungry	○	○	○	○	○
Uplifted	○	○	○	○	○
Creative	○	○	○	○	○

Ratings ☆ ☆ ☆ ☆ ☆

Strain

Grower _____   Date _____

Acquired _____ $ _____

Indica	Hybrid	Sativa

☐ Flower   ☐ Edible   ☐ Concentrate

Symptoms Relieved

_____

_____

_____

_____

_____

Sweet
Fruity   Floral
Sour   Spicy
Earthy   Herbal
Woodsy

Notes

_____

_____

_____

_____

_____

_____

Effects	Strength				
Peaceful	○	○	○	○	○
Sleepy	○	○	○	○	○
Pain Relief	○	○	○	○	○
Hungry	○	○	○	○	○
Uplifted	○	○	○	○	○
Creative	○	○	○	○	○

Ratings ☆ ☆ ☆ ☆ ☆

Strain

Grower _____ Date _____

Acquired _____ $ _____

Indica	Hybrid	Sativa

☐ Flower   ☐ Edible   ☐ Concentrate

Symptoms Relieved

_____
_____
_____
_____

Sweet

Fruity   Floral

Sour   Spicy

Earthy   Herbal

Woodsy

Notes

_____
_____
_____
_____
_____
_____

Effects	Strength				
Peaceful	○	○	○	○	○
Sleepy	○	○	○	○	○
Pain Relief	○	○	○	○	○
Hungry	○	○	○	○	○
Uplifted	○	○	○	○	○
Creative	○	○	○	○	○

Ratings ☆ ☆ ☆ ☆ ☆

Strain

Grower ....   Date ....

Acquired .... $ ....

Indica	Hybrid	Sativa

☐ Flower   ☐ Edible   ☐ Concentrate

Symptoms Relieved

....

....

....

....

Sweet

Fruity   Floral

Sour   Spicy

Earthy   Herbal

Woodsy

Notes

....

....

....

....

....

....

Effects	Strength				
Peaceful	○	○	○	○	○
Sleepy	○	○	○	○	○
Pain Relief	○	○	○	○	○
Hungry	○	○	○	○	○
Uplifted	○	○	○	○	○
Creative	○	○	○	○	○

Ratings ☆ ☆ ☆ ☆ ☆

Strain

Grower _____   Date _____

Acquired _____ $ _____

Indica	Hybrid	Sativa

☐ Flower   ☐ Edible   ☐ Concentrate

Symptoms Relieved

_____

_____

_____

_____

Sweet
Fruity   Floral
Sour   Spicy
Earthy   Herbal
Woodsy

Notes

_____

_____

_____

_____

_____

Effects	Strength				
Peaceful	○	○	○	○	○
Sleepy	○	○	○	○	○
Pain Relief	○	○	○	○	○
Hungry	○	○	○	○	○
Uplifted	○	○	○	○	○
Creative	○	○	○	○	○

Ratings ☆ ☆ ☆ ☆ ☆

Strain

Grower _____   Date _____

Acquired _____ $ _____

Indica	Hybrid	Sativa

☐ Flower   ☐ Edible   ☐ Concentrate

Symptoms Relieved

_____

_____

_____

_____

Sweet

Fruity   Floral

Sour   Spicy

Earthy   Herbal

Woodsy

Notes

_____

_____

_____

_____

_____

_____

Effects	Strength				
Peaceful	○	○	○	○	○
Sleepy	○	○	○	○	○
Pain Relief	○	○	○	○	○
Hungry	○	○	○	○	○
Uplifted	○	○	○	○	○
Creative	○	○	○	○	○

Ratings ☆ ☆ ☆ ☆ ☆

Strain

Grower _____   Date _____

Acquired _____ $ _____

Indica	Hybrid	Sativa

☐ Flower   ☐ Edible   ☐ Concentrate

Symptoms Relieved

_____

_____

_____

_____

Sweet
Fruity   Floral
Sour   Spicy
Earthy   Herbal
Woodsy

Notes

_____

_____

_____

_____

_____

_____

Effects	Strength				
Peaceful	○	○	○	○	○
Sleepy	○	○	○	○	○
Pain Relief	○	○	○	○	○
Hungry	○	○	○	○	○
Uplifted	○	○	○	○	○
Creative	○	○	○	○	○

Ratings ☆ ☆ ☆ ☆ ☆

Strain

Grower _____   Date _____

Acquired _____ $ _____

Indica	Hybrid	Sativa

☐ Flower   ☐ Edible   ☐ Concentrate

Symptoms Relieved

_____

_____

_____

_____

_____

Sweet

Fruity   Floral

Sour   Spicy

Earthy   Herbal

Woodsy

Notes

_____

_____

_____

_____

_____

Effects	Strength				
Peaceful	○	○	○	○	○
Sleepy	○	○	○	○	○
Pain Relief	○	○	○	○	○
Hungry	○	○	○	○	○
Uplifted	○	○	○	○	○
Creative	○	○	○	○	○

Ratings ☆ ☆ ☆ ☆ ☆

Strain

Grower _____   Date _____

Acquired _____ $ _____

Indica	Hybrid	Sativa

☐ Flower   ☐ Edible   ☐ Concentrate

Symptoms Relieved

_____

_____

_____

_____

Sweet

Fruity   Floral

Sour   Spicy

Earthy   Herbal

Woodsy

Notes

_____

_____

_____

_____

_____

_____

Effects	Strength				
Peaceful	○	○	○	○	○
Sleepy	○	○	○	○	○
Pain Relief	○	○	○	○	○
Hungry	○	○	○	○	○
Uplifted	○	○	○	○	○
Creative	○	○	○	○	○

Ratings ☆ ☆ ☆ ☆ ☆

Strain

Grower _____   Date _____

Acquired _____ $ _____

| Indica | Hybrid | Sativa |

☐ Flower   ☐ Edible   ☐ Concentrate

Symptoms Relieved

_____
_____
_____
_____

Sweet
Fruity   Floral
Sour   Spicy
Earthy   Herbal
Woodsy

Notes

_____
_____
_____
_____
_____
_____

Effects	Strength				
Peaceful	○	○	○	○	○
Sleepy	○	○	○	○	○
Pain Relief	○	○	○	○	○
Hungry	○	○	○	○	○
Uplifted	○	○	○	○	○
Creative	○	○	○	○	○

Ratings ☆ ☆ ☆ ☆ ☆

Strain

Grower _____   Date _____

Acquired _____ $ _____

| Indica | Hybrid | Sativa |

☐ Flower   ☐ Edible   ☐ Concentrate

Symptoms Relieved

_____
_____
_____
_____

Sweet
Fruity
Floral
Sour
Spicy
Earthy
Herbal
Woodsy

Notes

_____
_____
_____
_____
_____
_____

Effects	Strength				
Peaceful	○	○	○	○	○
Sleepy	○	○	○	○	○
Pain Relief	○	○	○	○	○
Hungry	○	○	○	○	○
Uplifted	○	○	○	○	○
Creative	○	○	○	○	○

Ratings ☆ ☆ ☆ ☆ ☆

Strain

Grower _____   Date _____

Acquired _____ $ _____

Indica	Hybrid	Sativa

☐ Flower   ☐ Edible   ☐ Concentrate

Symptoms Relieved

_____

_____

_____

_____

Sweet

Fruity   Floral

Sour   Spicy

Earthy   Herbal

Woodsy

Notes

_____

_____

_____

_____

_____

Effects	Strength				
Peaceful	○	○	○	○	○
Sleepy	○	○	○	○	○
Pain Relief	○	○	○	○	○
Hungry	○	○	○	○	○
Uplifted	○	○	○	○	○
Creative	○	○	○	○	○

Ratings ☆ ☆ ☆ ☆ ☆

Strain

Grower _____   Date _____

Acquired _____ $ _____

| Indica | Hybrid | Sativa |

☐ Flower   ☐ Edible   ☐ Concentrate

Symptoms Relieved

_____

_____

_____

_____

Sweet

Fruity   Floral

Sour   Spicy

Earthy   Herbal

Woodsy

Notes

_____

_____

_____

_____

_____

_____

Effects	Strength
Peaceful	○ ○ ○ ○ ○
Sleepy	○ ○ ○ ○ ○
Pain Relief	○ ○ ○ ○ ○
Hungry	○ ○ ○ ○ ○
Uplifted	○ ○ ○ ○ ○
Creative	○ ○ ○ ○ ○

Ratings ☆ ☆ ☆ ☆ ☆

Strain

Grower _____ Date _____

Acquired _____ $ _____

Indica	Hybrid	Sativa

☐ Flower ☐ Edible ☐ Concentrate

Symptoms Relieved

_____

_____

_____

_____

Sweet
Fruity   Floral
Sour   Spicy
Earthy   Herbal
Woodsy

Notes

_____

_____

_____

_____

_____

_____

Effects	Strength				
Peaceful	○	○	○	○	○
Sleepy	○	○	○	○	○
Pain Relief	○	○	○	○	○
Hungry	○	○	○	○	○
Uplifted	○	○	○	○	○
Creative	○	○	○	○	○

Ratings ☆ ☆ ☆ ☆ ☆

Strain

Grower _____ Date _____

Acquired _____ $ _____

Indica	Hybrid	Sativa

☐ Flower ☐ Edible ☐ Concentrate

Symptoms Relieved

_____

_____

_____

_____

Sweet

Fruity   Floral

Sour   Spicy

Earthy   Herbal

Woodsy

Notes

_____

_____

_____

_____

_____

_____

Effects	Strength				
Peaceful	○	○	○	○	○
Sleepy	○	○	○	○	○
Pain Relief	○	○	○	○	○
Hungry	○	○	○	○	○
Uplifted	○	○	○	○	○
Creative	○	○	○	○	○

Ratings ☆ ☆ ☆ ☆ ☆

Strain

Grower _____ Date _____

Acquired _____ $ _____

| Indica | Hybrid | Sativa |

☐ Flower ☐ Edible ☐ Concentrate

Symptoms Relieved

_____

_____

_____

_____

_____

Sweet

Fruity   Floral

Sour   Spicy

Earthy   Herbal

Woodsy

Notes

_____

_____

_____

_____

_____

_____

Effects	Strength
Peaceful	○ ○ ○ ○ ○
Sleepy	○ ○ ○ ○ ○
Pain Relief	○ ○ ○ ○ ○
Hungry	○ ○ ○ ○ ○
Uplifted	○ ○ ○ ○ ○
Creative	○ ○ ○ ○ ○

Ratings ☆ ☆ ☆ ☆ ☆

Strain

Grower _____ Date _____

Acquired _____ $ _____

Indica	Hybrid	Sativa

☐ Flower   ☐ Edible   ☐ Concentrate

Symptoms Relieved

_____

_____

_____

_____

_____

Sweet

Fruity   Floral

Sour   Spicy

Earthy   Herbal

Woodsy

Notes

_____

_____

_____

_____

_____

_____

Effects	Strength
Peaceful	○ ○ ○ ○ ○
Sleepy	○ ○ ○ ○ ○
Pain Relief	○ ○ ○ ○ ○
Hungry	○ ○ ○ ○ ○
Uplifted	○ ○ ○ ○ ○
Creative	○ ○ ○ ○ ○

Ratings ☆ ☆ ☆ ☆ ☆

Strain

Grower _____ Date _____

Acquired _____ $ _____

| Indica | Hybrid | Sativa |

☐ Flower   ☐ Edible   ☐ Concentrate

Symptoms Relieved

_____
_____
_____
_____

Sweet
Fruity   Floral
Sour   Spicy
Earthy   Herbal
Woodsy

Notes

_____
_____
_____
_____
_____
_____

Effects	Strength				
Peaceful	○	○	○	○	○
Sleepy	○	○	○	○	○
Pain Relief	○	○	○	○	○
Hungry	○	○	○	○	○
Uplifted	○	○	○	○	○
Creative	○	○	○	○	○

Ratings ☆ ☆ ☆ ☆ ☆

Strain

Grower _____   Date _____

Acquired _____ $ _____

Indica	Hybrid	Sativa

☐ Flower   ☐ Edible   ☐ Concentrate

Symptoms Relieved

_____

_____

_____

_____

_____

Sweet
Fruity   Floral
Sour   Spicy
Earthy   Herbal
Woodsy

Notes

_____

_____

_____

_____

_____

_____

_____

Effects	Strength				
Peaceful	○	○	○	○	○
Sleepy	○	○	○	○	○
Pain Relief	○	○	○	○	○
Hungry	○	○	○	○	○
Uplifted	○	○	○	○	○
Creative	○	○	○	○	○

Ratings ☆ ☆ ☆ ☆ ☆

Strain

Grower _____ Date _____

Acquired _____ $ _____

Indica	Hybrid	Sativa

☐ Flower ☐ Edible ☐ Concentrate

Symptoms Relieved

_____

_____

_____

_____

Sweet
Fruity   Floral
Sour   Spicy
Earthy   Herbal
Woodsy

Notes

_____

_____

_____

_____

_____

Effects	Strength				
Peaceful	○	○	○	○	○
Sleepy	○	○	○	○	○
Pain Relief	○	○	○	○	○
Hungry	○	○	○	○	○
Uplifted	○	○	○	○	○
Creative	○	○	○	○	○

Ratings ☆ ☆ ☆ ☆ ☆

Strain

Grower _____   Date _____

Acquired _____ $ _____

Indica	Hybrid	Sativa

☐ Flower   ☐ Edible   ☐ Concentrate

Symptoms Relieved

_____

_____

_____

_____

_____

Sweet
Fruity   Floral
Sour   Spicy
Earthy   Herbal
Woodsy

Notes

_____

_____

_____

_____

_____

_____

Effects	Strength				
Peaceful	○	○	○	○	○
Sleepy	○	○	○	○	○
Pain Relief	○	○	○	○	○
Hungry	○	○	○	○	○
Uplifted	○	○	○	○	○
Creative	○	○	○	○	○

Ratings ☆ ☆ ☆ ☆ ☆

Strain

Grower _____ Date _____

Acquired _____ $ _____

Indica	Hybrid	Sativa

☐ Flower ☐ Edible ☐ Concentrate

Symptoms Relieved

_____

_____

_____

_____

_____

Sweet

Fruity   Floral

Sour   Spicy

Earthy   Herbal

Woodsy

Notes

_____

_____

_____

_____

_____

_____

Effects	Strength				
Peaceful	○	○	○	○	○
Sleepy	○	○	○	○	○
Pain Relief	○	○	○	○	○
Hungry	○	○	○	○	○
Uplifted	○	○	○	○	○
Creative	○	○	○	○	○

Ratings ☆ ☆ ☆ ☆ ☆

Strain

Grower _____ Date _____

Acquired _____ $ _____

Indica	Hybrid	Sativa

☐ Flower ☐ Edible ☐ Concentrate

Symptoms Relieved

_____
_____
_____
_____
_____

Sweet
Fruity
Floral
Sour
Spicy
Earthy
Herbal
Woodsy

Notes

_____
_____
_____
_____
_____
_____

Effects	Strength				
Peaceful	○	○	○	○	○
Sleepy	○	○	○	○	○
Pain Relief	○	○	○	○	○
Hungry	○	○	○	○	○
Uplifted	○	○	○	○	○
Creative	○	○	○	○	○

Ratings ☆ ☆ ☆ ☆ ☆

Strain

Grower _____ Date _____

Acquired _____ $ _____

| Indica | Hybrid | Sativa |

☐ Flower ☐ Edible ☐ Concentrate

Symptoms Relieved

_____

_____

_____

_____

_____

Sweet
Fruity   Floral
Sour   Spicy
Earthy   Herbal
Woodsy

Notes

_____

_____

_____

_____

_____

_____

Effects	Strength
Peaceful	○ ○ ○ ○ ○
Sleepy	○ ○ ○ ○ ○
Pain Relief	○ ○ ○ ○ ○
Hungry	○ ○ ○ ○ ○
Uplifted	○ ○ ○ ○ ○
Creative	○ ○ ○ ○ ○

Ratings ☆ ☆ ☆ ☆ ☆

Strain

Grower _____   Date _____

Acquired _____ $ _____

Indica	Hybrid	Sativa

☐ Flower   ☐ Edible   ☐ Concentrate

Symptoms Relieved

_____

_____

_____

_____

_____

Sweet · Fruity · Floral · Sour · Spicy · Earthy · Herbal · Woodsy

Notes

_____

_____

_____

_____

_____

_____

_____

Effects	Strength				
Peaceful	○	○	○	○	○
Sleepy	○	○	○	○	○
Pain Relief	○	○	○	○	○
Hungry	○	○	○	○	○
Uplifted	○	○	○	○	○
Creative	○	○	○	○	○

Ratings ☆ ☆ ☆ ☆ ☆

Strain

Grower _____ Date _____

Acquired _____ $ _____

Indica	Hybrid	Sativa

☐ Flower   ☐ Edible   ☐ Concentrate

Symptoms Relieved

_____

_____

_____

_____

Sweet
Fruity   Floral
Sour   Spicy
Earthy   Herbal
Woodsy

Notes

_____

_____

_____

_____

_____

_____

Effects	Strength				
Peaceful	○	○	○	○	○
Sleepy	○	○	○	○	○
Pain Relief	○	○	○	○	○
Hungry	○	○	○	○	○
Uplifted	○	○	○	○	○
Creative	○	○	○	○	○

Ratings ☆ ☆ ☆ ☆ ☆

Strain

Grower _____   Date _____

Acquired _____ $ _____

| Indica | Hybrid | Sativa |

☐ Flower   ☐ Edible   ☐ Concentrate

Symptoms Relieved

_____

_____

_____

_____

_____

Sweet
Fruity
Floral
Sour
Spicy
Earthy
Herbal
Woodsy

Notes

_____

_____

_____

_____

_____

_____

Effects	Strength
Peaceful	○ ○ ○ ○ ○
Sleepy	○ ○ ○ ○ ○
Pain Relief	○ ○ ○ ○ ○
Hungry	○ ○ ○ ○ ○
Uplifted	○ ○ ○ ○ ○
Creative	○ ○ ○ ○ ○

Ratings ☆ ☆ ☆ ☆ ☆

Strain

Grower _____ Date _____

Acquired _____ $ _____

| Indica | Hybrid | Sativa |

☐ Flower ☐ Edible ☐ Concentrate

Symptoms Relieved

_____

_____

_____

_____

_____

Sweet

Fruity   Floral

Sour   Spicy

Earthy   Herbal

Woodsy

Notes

_____

_____

_____

_____

_____

_____

Effects	Strength				
Peaceful	○	○	○	○	○
Sleepy	○	○	○	○	○
Pain Relief	○	○	○	○	○
Hungry	○	○	○	○	○
Uplifted	○	○	○	○	○
Creative	○	○	○	○	○

Ratings ☆ ☆ ☆ ☆ ☆

Strain

Grower _____ Date _____

Acquired _____ $ _____

Indica	Hybrid	Sativa

☐ Flower ☐ Edible ☐ Concentrate

Symptoms Relieved

_____
_____
_____
_____

Sweet
Fruity   Floral
Sour   Spicy
Earthy   Herbal
Woodsy

Notes

_____
_____
_____
_____
_____
_____

Effects	Strength				
Peaceful	○	○	○	○	○
Sleepy	○	○	○	○	○
Pain Relief	○	○	○	○	○
Hungry	○	○	○	○	○
Uplifted	○	○	○	○	○
Creative	○	○	○	○	○

Ratings ☆ ☆ ☆ ☆ ☆

Strain

Grower _____   Date _____

Acquired _____ $ _____

Indica	Hybrid	Sativa

☐ Flower   ☐ Edible   ☐ Concentrate

Symptoms Relieved

_____
_____
_____
_____
_____

Sweet

Fruity   Floral

Sour   Spicy

Earthy   Herbal

Woodsy

Notes

_____
_____
_____
_____
_____
_____
_____

Effects	Strength				
Peaceful	○	○	○	○	○
Sleepy	○	○	○	○	○
Pain Relief	○	○	○	○	○
Hungry	○	○	○	○	○
Uplifted	○	○	○	○	○
Creative	○	○	○	○	○

Ratings ☆ ☆ ☆ ☆ ☆

Strain

Grower _____   Date _____

Acquired _____ $ _____

| Indica | Hybrid | Sativa |

☐ Flower   ☐ Edible   ☐ Concentrate

Symptoms Relieved

_____

_____

_____

_____

_____

Sweet

Fruity   Floral

Sour   Spicy

Earthy   Herbal

Woodsy

Notes

_____

_____

_____

_____

_____

_____

Effects	Strength				
Peaceful	○	○	○	○	○
Sleepy	○	○	○	○	○
Pain Relief	○	○	○	○	○
Hungry	○	○	○	○	○
Uplifted	○	○	○	○	○
Creative	○	○	○	○	○

Ratings ☆ ☆ ☆ ☆ ☆

Strain

Grower _____   Date _____

Acquired _____ $ _____

Indica	Hybrid	Sativa

☐ Flower ☐ Edible ☐ Concentrate

Symptoms Relieved

_____

_____

_____

_____

Sweet
Fruity   Floral
Sour   Spicy
Earthy   Herbal
Woodsy

Notes

_____

_____

_____

_____

_____

_____

Effects	Strength				
Peaceful	○	○	○	○	○
Sleepy	○	○	○	○	○
Pain Relief	○	○	○	○	○
Hungry	○	○	○	○	○
Uplifted	○	○	○	○	○
Creative	○	○	○	○	○

Ratings ☆ ☆ ☆ ☆ ☆

Strain

Grower _____   Date _____

Acquired _____ $ _____

| Indica | Hybrid | Sativa |

☐ Flower   ☐ Edible   ☐ Concentrate

Symptoms Relieved

_____

_____

_____

_____

Sweet
Fruity   Floral
Sour   Spicy
Earthy   Herbal
Woodsy

Notes

_____

_____

_____

_____

_____

_____

Effects	Strength				
Peaceful	○	○	○	○	○
Sleepy	○	○	○	○	○
Pain Relief	○	○	○	○	○
Hungry	○	○	○	○	○
Uplifted	○	○	○	○	○
Creative	○	○	○	○	○

Ratings ☆ ☆ ☆ ☆ ☆

Strain

Grower _____   Date _____

Acquired _____ $ _____

Indica	Hybrid	Sativa

☐ Flower   ☐ Edible   ☐ Concentrate

Symptoms Relieved

_____

_____

_____

_____

Sweet

Fruity   Floral

Sour   Spicy

Earthy   Herbal

Woodsy

Notes

_____

_____

_____

_____

_____

Effects	Strength				
Peaceful	○	○	○	○	○
Sleepy	○	○	○	○	○
Pain Relief	○	○	○	○	○
Hungry	○	○	○	○	○
Uplifted	○	○	○	○	○
Creative	○	○	○	○	○

Ratings ☆ ☆ ☆ ☆ ☆

Strain

Grower _____ Date _____

Acquired _____ $ _____

| Indica | Hybrid | Sativa |

☐ Flower ☐ Edible ☐ Concentrate

Symptoms Relieved

_____

_____

_____

_____

_____

Sweet

Fruity   Floral

Sour   Spicy

Earthy   Herbal

Woodsy

Notes

_____

_____

_____

_____

_____

_____

Effects	Strength				
Peaceful	○	○	○	○	○
Sleepy	○	○	○	○	○
Pain Relief	○	○	○	○	○
Hungry	○	○	○	○	○
Uplifted	○	○	○	○	○
Creative	○	○	○	○	○

Ratings ☆ ☆ ☆ ☆ ☆

Strain

Grower _____ Date _____

Acquired _____ $ _____

| Indica | Hybrid | Sativa |

☐ Flower ☐ Edible ☐ Concentrate

Symptoms Relieved

_____
_____
_____
_____

Sweet
Fruity / Floral
Sour / Spicy
Earthy / Herbal
Woodsy

Notes

_____
_____
_____
_____
_____
_____
_____

Effects	Strength				
Peaceful	○	○	○	○	○
Sleepy	○	○	○	○	○
Pain Relief	○	○	○	○	○
Hungry	○	○	○	○	○
Uplifted	○	○	○	○	○
Creative	○	○	○	○	○

Ratings ☆ ☆ ☆ ☆ ☆

Strain

Grower _____   Date _____

Acquired _____ $ _____

Indica	Hybrid	Sativa

☐ Flower   ☐ Edible   ☐ Concentrate

Symptoms Relieved

_____

_____

_____

_____

Sweet

Fruity   Floral

Sour   Spicy

Earthy   Herbal

Woodsy

Notes

_____

_____

_____

_____

_____

_____

Effects	Strength				
Peaceful	○	○	○	○	○
Sleepy	○	○	○	○	○
Pain Relief	○	○	○	○	○
Hungry	○	○	○	○	○
Uplifted	○	○	○	○	○
Creative	○	○	○	○	○

Ratings ☆ ☆ ☆ ☆ ☆

Strain

Grower _____ Date _____

Acquired _____ $ _____

Indica	Hybrid	Sativa

☐ Flower ☐ Edible ☐ Concentrate

Symptoms Relieved

_____

_____

_____

_____

Sweet
Fruity   Floral
Sour   Spicy
Earthy   Herbal
Woodsy

Notes

_____

_____

_____

_____

_____

Effects	Strength				
Peaceful	○	○	○	○	○
Sleepy	○	○	○	○	○
Pain Relief	○	○	○	○	○
Hungry	○	○	○	○	○
Uplifted	○	○	○	○	○
Creative	○	○	○	○	○

Ratings ☆ ☆ ☆ ☆ ☆

Strain

Grower _____   Date _____

Acquired _____ $ _____

Indica	Hybrid	Sativa

☐ Flower   ☐ Edible   ☐ Concentrate

Symptoms Relieved

_____

_____

_____

_____

_____

Sweet

Fruity   Floral

Sour   Spicy

Earthy   Herbal

Woodsy

Notes

_____

_____

_____

_____

_____

_____

Effects	Strength				
Peaceful	○	○	○	○	○
Sleepy	○	○	○	○	○
Pain Relief	○	○	○	○	○
Hungry	○	○	○	○	○
Uplifted	○	○	○	○	○
Creative	○	○	○	○	○

Ratings ☆ ☆ ☆ ☆ ☆

Strain

Grower _____   Date _____

Acquired _____ $ _____

Indica	Hybrid	Sativa

☐ Flower   ☐ Edible   ☐ Concentrate

Symptoms Relieved

_____

_____

_____

_____

Sweet

Fruity   Floral

Sour   Spicy

Earthy   Herbal

Woodsy

Notes

_____

_____

_____

_____

_____

_____

Effects	Strength				
Peaceful	○	○	○	○	○
Sleepy	○	○	○	○	○
Pain Relief	○	○	○	○	○
Hungry	○	○	○	○	○
Uplifted	○	○	○	○	○
Creative	○	○	○	○	○

Ratings ☆ ☆ ☆ ☆ ☆

Strain

Grower _____   Date _____

Acquired _____ $ _____

Indica	Hybrid	Sativa

☐ Flower   ☐ Edible   ☐ Concentrate

Symptoms Relieved

_____
_____
_____
_____

Sweet
Fruity   Floral
Sour   Spicy
Earthy   Herbal
Woodsy

Notes

_____
_____
_____
_____
_____
_____

Effects	Strength				
Peaceful	○	○	○	○	○
Sleepy	○	○	○	○	○
Pain Relief	○	○	○	○	○
Hungry	○	○	○	○	○
Uplifted	○	○	○	○	○
Creative	○	○	○	○	○

Ratings ☆ ☆ ☆ ☆ ☆

Made in the USA
Monee, IL
16 July 2021